HIIT Workouts

Get HIIT Fit - Fast-track Your Way To A Shredded Super-fit New You With HIIT Workouts (HIIT training, high intensity interval training)

Table of Contents

Contents

Introduction

So, you've been following your workout program rigorously and running long distances, but you're finding that you still can't get that belly fat to budge. You try doing more and more cardio only to find that you start losing muscle! Your dream is slipping away and you need a new tool to help you get that nice toned body you promised yourself. You want to get your body fat to back off. But you want your muscles to remain. You want to look like those other people at the gym. How do they do it? . . .

If this is your predicament, welcome to the world of High Intensity Interval Training (HIIT). HIIT is the solution that you need to strip off body fat while actually adding quality, lean muscle mass.

High Intensity Interval Training (HIIT) is an advanced cardio training system that is all about burning as many calories as possible in as little time as possible while still keeping muscle tissue! It is achieved through short, but very intense, bursts of exercise performed at a maximum effort level with short recovery or low intensity periods in between. HIIT can be applied to many different exercises such as cycling, running, skipping, even calisthenics or weight training.

Benefits include:

1) Maximum fat loss.
2) Very little time required.
3) No equipment necessary.
4) Do it anywhere.
5) Lose weight, not muscle.

In this book we will show you how to HIIT your way to a better body. You will learn to utilize principles of HIIT to put together your own workout using the most effective exercises ever devised. There are also some powerful fat burning HIIT style example workouts to try. We will also walk you through safety so you don't hurt yourself while you're burning all those calories. First though, we need to understand the benefits and the misconceptions regarding HIIT...

Chapter 1

Why HIIT It?

Who Is Azumi Tabata?

HIIT all began with the Japanese Olympic Speed Skating Team. The Head Coach, Irisawa Koichi, created a High Intensity Interval Training Workout for his skaters. This consisted of 8 rounds. Each round was 20 seconds of intense work using a cycling ergometer followed by 10 seconds of rest. Koichi had one of his training coaches, Azumi Tabata, analyze the effectiveness of this workout using scientific methods. This is where the Tabata protocol (which HIIT training is based on) came about. Although Tabata didn't actually invent the training method, but because of widespread interest in his findings the workout was named after him. Tabata's studies showed his subjects producing impressive results that make traditional (steady state) cardio seem ineffective by comparison. The system claimed worldwide interest and HIIT style training (based on Azumi Tabata's research) has now become one of the most popular ways to train for a number of good reasons...

Benefits of HIIT Training

Efficiency:

Tabata found that this workout was extremely effective when it comes to burning a lot of calories in very little time (even just 5-10 minutes per day). It is, therefore, a very time efficient method of fat-burning and more effective for fat loss in time taken than steady state cardio. If you value your time and don't have much to spare for training then HIIT can be very handy.

The After burn Effect:

When Tabata did his experiments he found that subjects worked close to what is called VO2 max or the maximum oxygen the body uses in exercise. The more your muscles have to work the more the body uses. High intensity work like this means that the body has what is called an after burn where metabolism increases. This means that your body not only burns a lot of fat during exercise but also you will burn more calories for at least 24 hours after the workout!

Retain Muscle Tissue:

One problem encountered by folks doing cardio is that with a long time spent doing steady state cardio they may lose weight but they may lose significant muscle mass in the process. Just take a look at the difference between sprinters and long distance runners. Sprinters look muscular and sinewy. Long distance runners have lost a lot more muscle. So if you want to really change your shape and not just become smaller and yet keep your belly fat then HIIT is the way to do it right. In addition, high intensity cardio in the form of sprint work can actually add mass to the quadriceps.

Your Health:

HIIT training brings benefits in the areas of blood pressure, sensitivity to insulin, the cardiovascular system, and aerobic and anaerobic systems. Tabata's results showed an increase in anaerobic fitness by up to 28%. His subjects had stronger hearts and could perform faster and for longer after training. If you want to not only look strong and healthy but BE strong and healthy, you have simply got to HIIT it.

Versatility:

The principles of HIIT can be applied without any equipment and therefore can be done anywhere, including outside in the fresh air down at the local park. Keeping your knees high or performing burpies, jumping jacks, pushups or jumping lunges at high intensity can all get your heart rate up high. And weight training exercises can be given the HIIT treatment by making adjustments to the rep and rest schemes.

Misconceptions about HIIT training

1) Longer Training is Better Training

You don't need 60 or even 30 minutes to have a great HIIT workout The main principle behind High Intensity Training is that you go all out and push yourself to your limit periodically throughout the workout, even if it is only for a short time like 5-10 minutes. This means 2 minutes of steady state exercise to warm up, working at about 50% of your maximum effort. Next 20 seconds of all out effort, followed by 10 seconds of rest. Repeat the 20 and 10 second intervals 7 more times and then finish with another 2 minutes of steady state at half of your maximum effort. Doing that to your maximum ability will give your body more added value than 5 x more time spent on steady state cardio.

2) All Exercises are Well Suited for HIIT Training

Not all exercises are adequate for HIIT. To achieve real high intensity, aim to use full body movements that will tax your cardiovascular system, and build strength endurance, like kettle swings or sprints. Bicep curls or triceps extensions will only target one body part and will not achieve the effect of HIIT training. The best weight training movements are compound exercises that work multiple body parts. A good rule to follow is can you hold a conversation while you are doing it? If so, then you're not working hard enough.

3) HIIT Training will Bulk You Up

HIIT training will burn fat but let you keep the muscle you already have. To obtain more bulk you must do bodybuilding training. But exercises like swings or clean and pressing a heavy kettlebell or snatching a heavy dumbbell are good whole body exercises and can be used for HIIT training but these exercises can also build muscle. For bodybuilders who want a lower body fat percentage, HIIT training is perfect to burn it off and leave their hard earned bulk intact.

4) HIIT Alone Will Shed Fat

HIIT is indeed very efficient for burning lots of fat in a short time, and can also speed up your metabolism for a short time afterward. But this is no excuse to eat whatever you want, whenever you want. The fact is that your body is like a fuel tank and fat is the fuel. If you are taking in more than you are getting rid of then you will still have too much. Likewise, even if you are getting rid of it faster but you are still taking in too much, you won't get rid of it fast enough. This is why diet is an important component in a good HIIT training program.

Chapter 2

Safety and Establishing Base Fitness

HIIT is a very effective tool for burning fat. In some cases, however, it can be a little too effective, to the point where instead of just burning fat it just burns you! If you don't know what you're doing you can injure yourself, throw up or become a coronary risk. So, there are a few things you need to know before you decide to jump into HIIT training.

What's a sedentary lifestyle?

A sedentary lifestyle is a lifestyle where a person spends very little to zero time doing physical exercise. This is a serious concern if a person in this position wants to do HIIT training as they may be at risk of coronary disease.

Coronary disease is a blockage of one or more of the arteries that supply the heart with blood. This is usually because of hardening in the arteries. Symptoms include:

- Difficulty Breathing
- Chest pains or pains in other areas of the body such as your shoulder, back, neck or jaw.
- Nausea or vomiting
- Dizziness or light-headedness.
- Feeling of choking, indigestion or heartburn.
- A cold sweat.

If you were to experience any of these symptoms you would need immediate medical treatment from a professional as these can lead to heart failure.

Things like obesity, smoking, diabetes, abnormal cholesterol and hypertension will increase the risk of coronary further.

So for anybody with these conditions, before starting a HIIT training program it may be a very good idea to clear the air with a doctor or physician. It is also a good idea to establish a good foundation level of fitness before starting high intensity training. This can be done by taking part in regular (steady state) cardio consistently for 3 to 5 times per week at a challenging level. Doing this for several weeks will help your muscles adapt to take in more oxygen. It's important to develop muscle strength to avoid injury while performing various HIIT exercise routines. You will also need to understand proper use of weights when using weight-lifting exercises for this same reason.

Proper Use of Weights

There is the possibility for serious injury if weights are not handled carefully. Weights are heavy and they can do serious damage. To avoid this weights must be gripped correctly. There are three different kinds of grip you can use with dumbbells and bars; pronated (overhand with knuckles facing up), supinated (underhand with knuckles facing down) and mixed with one of each.

Your grip should be tight and closed so that your fingers and thumbs are all wrapped around the bar or dumbbell. An open grip where you leave your thumbs out is dangerous and you can lose the bar or dumbbell.

Always be careful to lock barbells after loading as weights can fall off one end of the barbell and send you flying sideways or leave a gaping hole in your wood floor. Always check these periodically in case they come loose or you forget to lock them. If loading a barbell from a bench or heightened platform, make sure to get somebody to help you take the weight off both sides evenly, at the same time.

Don't hold your breath while lifting weights. Breathe naturally. For an exercise like squats for example breathe out as you push to standing position and breathe in as you descend back down. This will help you to keep your blood pressure from getting too high and avoid causing injuries like hernia.

Just Add Water

During a workout it is important to drink plenty of water. This will help you to avoid hurting yourself but it will also make your muscles much stronger and will even help you gain muscle and lose fat more easily. So drink lots of it. Drink some before, some after and keep drinking through your workout when you get a chance.

Nutrition

Many who take part in high intensity interval training find that they achieve the best results when they eat healthy. In fact many folks achieve very little fat loss even when training very hard, simply because they eat whatever they want in the meantime. This is not what we want. If you want to achieve consistent fat loss and build muscle, you need to eat right.

Some good ideas are to eat multiple, small meals in a day (around six) as opposed to one large, pig out meal. Stick to lots of lean meats and vegetables and carbs that digest slowly.

Many also find that they have much better results with HIIT training when they do it on an empty stomach.

Chapter 3

Top HIIT Exercises

There are literally hundreds of exercises out there that you can apply to HIIT training and be used to burn some serious fat. You can keep it simple by using just a treadmill, a skipping rope, a bicycle or any cardio machine you may find at a gym, or you can put together mixed routines that change at each interval and throw in some dumbbells or a kettle bell and work muscles too.

To make sure that you get the full benefits of HIIT training you want to use your whole body throughout a workout to up that heart rate and get the after burn effect. For that reason we won't be discussing bicep curls or kickbacks. Instead, we will focus on compound exercises that get you closer to your VO2 max. In this chapter, we'll provide the technique for the best HIIT movements to burn fat and get super lean. Take the time to learn proper technique in order to avoid injuries while working out.

Upper body

Rows

Start standing with your dumbbells in your hands at your sides. Bend forward from the hips but keep your back straight! Allow the weight to hang down toward the ground in front of you. Pull your elbows back close to your waist from this position. At the top of the movement squeeze your back muscles together and then lower the weights again. Make sure your back is nearly parallel to the floor during this exercise. You want to work back muscles not your shoulders. You can use dumbbells or a single kettlebell or even a bar for this one. This will work your back and arms.

Pushups

Start lying face down on the floor with your hands next to your shoulders and your toes on the floor. Keeping your back and legs totally straight push your body off the floor until your arms are straight. Lower your body slowly to the floor by bending your elbows while keeping back and legs straight. Keep your elbows fairly close to your waist as you do this. If it is too hard then you can try keeping your knees on the floor as your body's pivot point instead of your feet. Regardless don't let your hips sag to the floor or stick your butt out to the sky. This will work your chest, shoulders and arms.

Lower Body

Dumbbell Squats

Stand with dumbbells at your sides in your hands. Place your feet at about the same distance apart as your hips and turn your toes slightly out. Slowly bend your knees while you push out your backside. Go as low as you can comfortably or to where your thighs become parallel to the ground. Push back up to starting position. Push through your heels not your toes; your heels should hold more of your weight. Don't let your back hunch forward at any point. Keep your backside stuck out as far as you can behind you. This can be done with a single kettlebell in front, a barbell in front resting across the upper arms or behind the neck resting across the shoulders.

Lunges

Start standing with dumbbells in your hands at your sides and your feet shoulder width. Step forward with one foot and bend that knee as you lower your body. Your other knee should almost touch the ground. Push with your front foot to stand up again and bring your back foot forward next to your other foot the same as your starting position. Repeat but swap sides. If this is too hard don't use any weights or you can increase them if you want to. Keep your back straight.

Core/Abs

Sit Ups

Start lying on your back, with your knees bent and your feet flat on the ground. Place your hands by your sides. Pull in your belly button so that your entire back gets to touch the ground and roll up until you are sitting upright. Reverse back down. You can put your feet under a couch or something that will achieve the same to stabilize yourself while you perform the sit up if it is too hard to do normally. You can also take one leg off the ground and put it up in the air if you want an extra challenge.

Leg Lifts

Lay on your back the same as with the sit ups. Keep your hands beside you, your feet together and your legs straight. Now, while keeping your legs straight, lift both of them so that they are at a right angle to the floor. Keep your back touching the floor. Lower your legs slowly back to the floor. If you have any strain in your lower back you can try putting your hands under your backside. If this is too hard you can lower one leg at a time or bend your knees so that your lower leg is parallel with the floor when raised. If it becomes too easy try lifting your upper back off the floor at the same time.

Compound Exercises

Burpees

Start in a standing position. No weights. Squat down and put your hands on the ground. Next jump your feet backward so that you're in the push up position. Jump them forward again into the squat position and then jump once on the spot and you are back at the start position. If this exercise is too hard you can try stepping back and forward instead of jumping. For an additional challenge try jumping onto a box or step and back down, rather than jumping on the spot. You can increase the height of the box or step.

Kettlebell / Dumbbell Swing

Start in a standing position with your feet out wide and toes slightly outward. You should be holding a kettle bell or dumbbell in front of you in both hands. Next bend your knees and push out your backside. Keep your back straight and your abs tight and swing the kettle back like you are trying to grab the wall behind you. Now stand, push your pelvis forward and swing the kettle with your arms straight until they are holding the kettle straight out in front of you at head height. You are not lifting with your arms. You should be using your hips and legs for the hard work. You will be doing this quite explosively and using momentum. Increase or decrease weights to vary the challenge.

Dumbbell Clean and Press

Start standing, feet shoulder width apart and two dumbbells on the ground in front of you. Keeping your back straight, bend your knees and hip joints and pick up the dumbbells with your arms straight. Start straightening your legs and pulling the weight from the ground. Move your pelvis forward and raise your shoulders and shrug them, using the momentum to pull the weight up as high as you can but keep it close to your body. Rotate your palms so they face up and your elbows so they point forward and bring your body under the weights so they sit at your shoulder level. Stand up and push the dumbbells over your head. Lower them back to the floor without hunching your back and keeping your pelvis back. Increase or decrease weight to vary the challenge. You can use a barbell for this exercise too.

Chapter 4

Constructing Your Workout

Here is where you create your own HIIT training program to get you ripped. The great thing about HIIT training is that it can be easily adapted to fit people of all levels of fitness or for people with health conditions. HIIT can be done using all manner of exercise such as running, cycling, swimming, cross-training and even weight training. To design a HIIT training program you simply need to have some good fat burning exercises that you know how to do properly, and to put them into a specified timeframe for how long your workout will take. You will have a number of rounds or time periods in your workout and you should decide how long they will be individually. These will include high intensity periods, periods of rest and a warm up and warm down that is moderately intense or half way between.

Your Program

Here is an example of what your program should look like:

2 minute warm up- A steady jog.

20 seconds high intensity kettlebell swinging (you can aim for a certain number of reps).

10 seconds rest.

20 seconds high intensity squats with a kettlebell.

10 seconds rest.

20 seconds high intensity burpees.

10 seconds rest.

20 seconds high intensity pushups.

10 seconds rest.

2 minute warm down- Steady jog.

This is modeled after the Tabata method of training and you will notice that it only amounts to a 4 minute workout in the end. However this is the same method that the Japanese Olympic Speed Skating Team used in their training. It is not for the faint of heart. This workout will absolutely destroy you. A good recommendation is to start by increasing the rest times in between to several minutes to give a body that doesn't belong to a pro athlete some time to regenerate it's energy for the next sprint. You can slowly decrease them in time for an added challenge. But the important part is that the 20 seconds be as intense as you can muster.

With this program you can slot in your selection of activities and select the intensity for yourself. You can work through the entire program on just a treadmill or cycle, or you can make the workout entirely out of compound weight training exercises. All you have to make sure of is that it consists of short bursts of intense activity followed by rest.

Note: Before starting this program it's a good idea to make sure you have plenty of water on hand as your body performs best when well hydrated. Drink continually throughout your workout during rest periods and also before and after you start. Lack of hydration can be dangerous but also the water will help you to gain muscle and lose fat and will also make you stronger during your workout. Finally make sure to lift weights in the correct way and be careful when loading weights to avoid injury.

This workout Timeframe can be adapted to suit any level of fitness. What is considered intense may be different for different people if weight and speed are the factors being compared. But when comparing how much effort goes in you want to say that at a workout's high point you are pushing yourself up to a good 90 percent of what you consider the hardest you can possibly go.

You can find out what this is by starting small and constantly setting goals to increase with each workout how high your intensity goes. You can also measure your heart rate to find out whether you are reaching your high zone with HIIT.

To do this there is a simple formula: 208- (age x 0.7) x 85 percent= high zone. You can use a good quality heart monitor to see whether you are reaching this intensity level. So long as you know you are going all out with a ten out of ten effort then you will be achieving high intensity.

Chapter Five

Final Word

High Intensity Interval Training will challenge every fiber of your self discipline. You will burn fat like never before and build and retain muscle that will pop from your body. Your performance will go up at any activity that requires short stints of go time. But more importantly you will learn self discipline and how to push yourself to your limit at anything. We hope that you will use HIIT to continue to push your limit and discover ever greater the power that you have to change your body and your life.

Sage Surefire

Subscribe to our list to get notified of new book releases from Sage Surefire. We notify you of new book releases, updates to the books, and when a book is given away free.

http://eepurl.com/bronjj

You'll like my other books.

Women Bodybuilding: Build a lean, sexy, toned, curvy body without getting bulky

http://www.amazon.com/gp/product/B00YB9SAN0?*Version*=1&*entries*=0

CrossFit Training: Build a lean, athletic, sexy body with fresh and exciting crossfit workouts

http://www.amazon.com/gp/product/B00Z14BENW?*Version*=1&*entries*=0

Building Muscle: Bullshit free secrets to building muscle

http://www.amazon.com/gp/product/B010INJBPS?*Version*=1&*entries*=0